HERBS FOR LIVER CLEANSING

Harnessing Nature's Healing Power, Unlocking The Secrets Detoxification Through Medicinal Remedies

DR. JEREMY ALLEY

Copyright © DR. JEREMY ALLEY 2024

All rights reserved. No part of this publication may be reproduced, distributed, or transmitted in any form or by any means, including photocopying, recording, or other electronic or mechanical methods, without the prior written permission of the author, except in the case of brief quotations embodied in critical reviews and certain other noncommercial uses permitted by copyright law.

Disclaimer:

The information provided in this book, is intended for general informational purposes only and should not be considered as professional advice.

The author has made every effort to ensure the accuracy of the information presented. However, readers are advised to consult with a qualified healthcare professional before attempting any herbal remedies or making significant changes to their wellness routine. Individual health conditions vary, and what may be suitable for one person may not be appropriate for another.

It is important to note that the author is not in any endorsement deal, partnership, or affiliation with any organization, brand, or company mentioned in this book. Any references to specific products or services are based on the author's personal experience or general knowledge and do not imply an endorsement or promotion of those products or services.

Contents

Overview

Herbal remedies have drawn a lot of interest in the field of holistic health because of their potential advantages in treating a range of medical issues. This book explores the use of herbal remedies, with a particular emphasis on their use in liver and blood cleaning. For individuals searching for sustainable and natural methods of maintaining their health, it is essential to comprehend the role that these herbal medicines play in enhancing general well-being.

About This Book

Welcome to a thorough investigation of herbal medicines designed to improve the health of your liver and blood. We must accept the abundance of natural resources available to us on this trip, as well as their capacity to aid the body's inherent cleansing processes. This section is a warm welcome to explore the potential of herbs to support ideal blood and liver function.

Concerning Herbal Treatments

Gaining a basic understanding of herbal remedies is essential before diving into specialized herbal solutions for liver and blood cleansing. For millennia, people from diverse cultures have used these plant-based, natural medicines for their medical benefits. Understanding the history, production processes, and mechanisms of action of herbal remedies paves the way for a deeper understanding of their capacity to enhance health and well-being.

The Value of Healthy Liver and Blood

Crucial to preserving the body's general health and internal balance are the liver and blood. Gaining an appreciation of these essential systems' relevance is essential to realizing the value of herbal remedies in promoting their optimal performance. The liver performs a variety of roles that affect several facets of health, including detoxification and nutritional digestion. Comparably, the blood acts as the body's lifeline, delivering oxygen, nutrition, and immune cells to every part of the body. Understanding how these systems work together emphasizes how important it is to give blood and liver health a priority for general health.

We shall examine a wide range of herbal medicines in the following sections of this book, each with special advantages for supporting liver and blood purification. With a focus on modern herbal ideas and tried-and-true traditional cures, this exploration hopes to arm readers with knowledge that can support their overall health.

Knowledge of the liver and blood

As the principal organ involved in detoxification, the liver of humans is vital to sustaining general health. It creates vital proteins, breaks down nutrients, and removes poisons from the blood. It is essential to know the complex interaction between the liver and blood to appreciate how important it is to preserve their optimal functions.

The Liver's Function in Detoxification

An important component of the body's detoxification process is the liver. Toxins are broken down and removed by it, preventing buildup and damage. The liver converts toxic substances into water-soluble compounds that can be expelled through urine or bile through several intricate metabolic processes. Protecting the body's general health by limiting the accumulation of dangerous compounds in the bloodstream is made possible by this detoxification process.

Blood's Roles in the Body

The blood circulates through a huge network of blood vessels, providing vital nutrients, oxygen, and hormones to numerous tissues and organs. Blood is the life power of the body. It is also essential for eliminating carbon dioxide and waste materials. Comprehending the diverse roles played by blood is vital in appreciating its importance in preserving general health and welfare.

Typical Problems with the Liver and Blood

Numerous variables can affect the liver's and blood's proper functioning, which can result in a variety of health problems. Liver disorders such as cirrhosis, hepatitis, and fatty liver disease can impair the liver's capacity to adequately detoxify the blood. Blood flow and functioning can be disrupted by blood-related illnesses, such as anemia, clotting disorders, and infections. It's critical to acknowledge these prevalent problems to put into practice practical measures that promote blood and liver health.

It is essential to take into account these basic characteristics of the liver and blood when we explore herbal remedies for liver and blood cleansing to understand the comprehensive approach needed to preserve a healthy circulatory and detoxification system.

CHAPTER ONE

ADVANTAGES OF HERBAL MEDICATIONS

Herbal remedies are widely known for their ability to support general health and wellness, especially for important organs like the liver and blood. Incorporating herbal medicines into one's healthcare practice has numerous inherent benefits, providing a natural and comprehensive approach to well-being. These remedies make use of the power of numerous plants, each of which has special qualities that aid in the liver and blood's renewal and purification.

The Potential Of Herbal Treatments

For ages, traditional medicine systems have relied heavily on herbs, and there is ample evidence of their effectiveness in promoting the health of the liver and blood. Numerous bioactive substances, including antioxidants, anti-inflammatory agents, and detoxifying components, are frequently found in herbal treatments. Together, these substances fight inflammation, oxidative stress, and the buildup of toxins in the blood and liver. Herbs' inherent power can help to reestablish equilibrium and improve the body's natural capacity to purge and cleanse essential fluids.

Benefits Compared To Conventional Therapies

Compared to traditional therapies, herbal remedies for liver and blood cleansing have fewer side effects, which is one of their main benefits. Herbs, when administered properly, tend to be kinder to the body than pharmaceutical drugs, which may have unintended side effects. In addition, herbal therapies frequently target the underlying causes of imbalances to provide a longer-lasting and more permanent remedy. This strategy differs from some traditional drugs, which could put more of an emphasis on managing symptoms than dealing with the underlying problems.

Herbal remedies' allure is also influenced by their holistic character. Herbal treatments consider the interdependence of all body systems, as opposed to focusing on isolating particular organs or symptoms. This all-encompassing strategy is consistent with the knowledge that good blood and liver health are not discrete issues, but rather are closely related to general well-being. Herbs enhance the body's natural homeostasis and promote balance, which might have a favorable effect on blood circulation and liver function.

A Comprehensive Approach To Blood And Liver Health

Herbal remedies take a multifaceted approach to liver and blood health by taking into account many facets of health. In addition to including herbal medicines, this holistic approach addresses food choices, stress management, and lifestyle issues. Herbs with liver-cleansing qualities include milk thistle, turmeric, burdock, and red clover; others, like dandelion, help with blood purification. When these herbs are included in a holistic health regimen, they work in concert to improve the body's capacity for detoxification and regeneration.

Beyond just relieving particular symptoms, herbal remedies for liver and blood cleansing have several advantages.

They represent a holistic outlook that acknowledges the many interrelationships found inside the body. Through the utilization of herbs, people can set off on a path to overall health and wellness, encouraging the best possible performance of two vital organ systems—the liver and the blood.

CHAPTER TWO

ESSENTIAL HERBS FOR CLEANING THE LIVER

An essential organ for detoxification and general health maintenance is the liver. Numerous herbs have been identified as having the ability to promote liver function and encourage cleaning. Milk thistle, known as nature's liver defender, is one such herb.

A substance found in milk thistle called silymarin is well-known for its antioxidant qualities, which support the liver's ability to repair damaged cells and protect it from poisons.

Another powerful plant for liver health is the dandelion root. This plant is highly valued for its ability to help the liver rid itself of toxic toxins. Dandelion root increases the production of bile, which aids with digestion and the breakdown of lipids. Its diuretic qualities aid in the removal of toxins from the liver and the body as a whole.

Turmeric is prized for its anti-inflammatory and antioxidant properties in addition to its vivid color and unique flavor. The major ingredient in turmeric, curcumin, has been researched for its ability to lessen oxidative stress and inflammation in the liver.

Turmeric As A Useful Supplement To Liver-Cleansing Regimens.

Artichokes have earned a spot in the field of liver health because of their ability to support liver function. It contains substances that help produce and move bile, such as silymarin and cynarin. Increased bile production improves nutrition absorption and digestion, which eventually benefits liver function.

Yellow dock is known for its ability to cleanse the liver as well as the blood. Anthraquinones, which are present in this herb, encourage the body to expel waste and induce bowel motions. Yellow dock helps the liver detoxify indirectly by promoting intestinal regularity.

Including these herbs in a comprehensive liver health regimen can help support the general health of this important organ. Before introducing new herbs or supplements, it is crucial to speak with a healthcare provider, particularly if there are any pre-existing medical conditions or concerns about possible prescription interactions.

CHAPTER THREE

HERBS TO PURIFY THE BLOOD

Maintaining general health requires blood purification, and many herbs have been shown to have extraordinary properties for blood cleansing and purification. These herbs are essential for clearing the blood of pollutants and poisons, which improves circulation and nurtures an individual's general health.

Burdock Root: Properties For Cleaning Blood

Burdock root is one famous herb known for its blood-cleansing qualities. For generations, burdock has been utilized in traditional medicine as a means of detoxifying the blood. It has substances that help the liver operate, which helps the bloodstream get rid of waste and contaminants. Burdock root also contains anti-inflammatory qualities, which adds to its potency in supporting blood health.

Red Clover: Increasing Blood Flow

Another herb that is notable for enhancing blood circulation is red clover. Compounds in this herb aid in blood vessel relaxation, promoting more fluid blood flow. Red clover helps the body move nutrients and oxygen more efficiently by improving circulation. This helps to keep the heart healthy generally and helps to purify the blood.

Echinacea: Strengthening Immune System for Healthy Blood

Though its ability to strengthen immunity is its most well-known benefit, echinacea also helps to keep blood healthy. Echinacea aids the body's defense against illnesses and viruses that could jeopardize the blood's purity by fortifying the immune system. Strong immune function promotes general health and helps the body's processes for cleansing blood.

Taking Licorice Root To Balance Blood Sugar

In addition to its sweet taste, licorice root has been shown to have the ability to stabilize blood sugar levels. Blood health as a whole may be impacted by fluctuations in blood sugar. The substances included in licorice root may aid in blood sugar regulation and circulatory stability. The fact that this herb is used in herbal therapies for blood purification highlights how different body processes are interdependent.

Garlic: Organic Blood Purifier

Garlic's sulfur-containing components, such as allicin, have earned it the reputation of being a natural blood cleaner. It has been demonstrated that these substances contain antioxidant and anti-inflammatory qualities, which help to purify blood. Garlic helps the liver eliminate impurities and keeps cholesterol levels in check, which further improves cardiovascular health and blood purity in general.

Including these herbs in a healthy, balanced diet can aid in the blood's natural cleaning processes. But, before making big dietary changes or adding new herbs, especially if you have pre-existing medical concerns or are on medication, it is imperative to speak with a healthcare provider.

CHAPTER FOUR

FUSING HERBAL COMPOSITES

The skill of making herbal blends is essential when using herbal medicines to cleanse the liver and purify the blood. Combinations of various herbs that have been carefully picked for their unique qualities that support the health of the liver and blood are known as herbal blends. Because of their well-known detoxifying properties, common herbs including milk thistle, burdock, and dandelion root are frequently included. Knowing the qualities of each plant and how they complement one another is essential to making a well-balanced and potent herbal combination.

The Combinatorial Effects Of Herbs

Enhancing the advantages of any individual herb in a blend depends on how well they work together. It's crucial to choose herbs for liver and blood cleansing that work well together to enhance overall organ function and encourage detoxification. Herbs with anti-inflammatory qualities, such as turmeric, can be used in conjunction with other herbs, such as artichoke leaf, which supports liver function. Herbalists and individuals can optimize the potential health benefits of the herbal combinations they develop by being aware of the synergistic effects.

Recipes For Herbal Tea To Support Blood And Liver Health

Herbal teas are a well-liked and entertaining way to use herbal remedies for blood and liver cleansing. Herbal teas are a convenient method to take a range of herbs that are known for their cleaning benefits, in addition to being hydrating.

Ginger, licorice root, and nettle are common constituents in liver and blood health teas. You can sip these teas all day long to help the body's natural detoxification processes moderately and consistently.

Extracts And Tinctures: Simple Dosage Choices

Tinctures and extracts provide simple dosage alternatives for individuals looking for a more concentrated and practical form of herbal treatment.

In tinctures, the active ingredients are extracted from botanicals with glycerin or alcohol. It is simple to incorporate this concentrated liquid into juice or water for consumption.

Herbal extracts, which come in a variety of forms, offer a powerful and efficient means of incorporating herbs that cleanse the liver and blood into a daily regimen. Those with hectic schedules can use these concentrated formulations since they enable precise and controlled dosing.

Effective herbal remedies for liver and blood cleansing involve the construction of herbal blends, knowledge of their synergistic effects, experimentation with herbal tea recipes, and incorporation of tinctures or extracts. Whether you like to take a potent tincture or a relaxing cup of herbal tea, the secret is to consistently and thoughtfully include these herbal medicines into a whole-person approach to health and wellbeing.

CHAPTER FIVE

INCLUDING HERBAL SOLUTIONS IN YOUR DAILY ROUTINE

Herbal remedies can be a helpful and comprehensive strategy for supporting liver and blood health when added to your everyday routine. For millennia, people from many different cultures have used herbs for their possible medical benefits. We'll look at a few of the herbs that are well-known for purifying the blood and liver in this part.

Dietary Guidelines For Blood And Liver Health

Making mindful food decisions is essential to supporting clean blood and preserving a healthy liver.

Some herbs are quite helpful in promoting these important organs.

For example, dandelion root has long been used to support liver function and is well known for its cleansing qualities. Another herb that has been shown to safeguard and enhance liver health by aiding in detoxification processes is milk thistle. We will explore the dietary guidelines in this area that can be used in conjunction with herbal remedies to achieve the best possible liver and blood health.

Modifications To Lifestyle For Long-Term Gains

Herbal medicines aid in blood and liver cleansing, but long-term benefits also depend on implementing permanent lifestyle modifications.

This entails forming healthful routines like cutting back on alcohol, steering clear of processed meals, and controlling stress.

This section will look at how these dietary adjustments combined with herbal remedies can promote liver and blood health in a whole new way.

Exercise's Effects On The Liver And Blood

Frequent physical activity provides numerous advantages for general health, including improved blood and liver function.

Frequent exercise promotes better blood circulation, which supports the liver's effective operation.

In addition, exercise maintains a healthy cardiovascular system and encourages the sweating out of impurities.

 In this section, we will look at how adding exercise to your regimen can work in conjunction with herbal remedies to provide a complete blood and liver cleansing regimen.

Herbal remedies can be used in conjunction with dietary modifications, lifestyle alterations, and consistent exercise to help people promote their liver and blood health as a whole.

It's crucial to remember that, for individualized advice and safety, you should always seek medical advice before making big changes to your health regimen.

CHAPTER SIX

SUCCESS STORIES AND CASE STUDIES

Experiences from everyday life offer important perspectives on the effectiveness of herbal remedies for blood and liver purification. This chapter includes case studies that show how people used herbal treatments to improve their blood and liver health. These accounts provide concrete illustrations of how herbal remedies have improved people's lives.

Actual Case Studies Of Herbal Remedies

This section explores more general real-world experiences of herbal remedies than just case studies. Readers will come across a variety of narratives, anecdotes, and testimonies from people who have made herbal treatments a regular part of their lives. These accounts add to a comprehensive knowledge of the usefulness and possible advantages of using herbal remedies for blood and liver cleansing.

Testimonials From People Who Have Profited From The Treatments

To emphasize the effectiveness of herbal treatments even more, this chapter gathers testimonies from people who have seen real results from adding these cures to their daily routines. These first-hand experiences attest to the beneficial effects of herbal therapies on blood and liver health, enticing readers to think about these all-natural methods for their health.

Through firsthand accounts and testimonies, readers will not only learn about herbal remedies for liver and blood purification but also acquire a sophisticated comprehension of their pragmatic uses as they peruse the book's pages.

CHAPTER SEVEN

AWARENESS AND ACCESSORIES

It's important to think about safety before starting a herbal journey for blood and liver cleansing. Certain plants are not good for everyone, and people react differently to different herbs. Individuals who already have liver disease should use caution and consult medical authorities.

Rather than being the only treatment, herbal therapies should be used in conjunction with a healthy lifestyle that includes regular exercise and a balanced diet.

Speaking With Medical Experts

Speaking with medical professionals is essential before beginning any herbal liver and blood cleansing program.

Based on a person's medical history, they can offer tailored guidance to make sure that selected herbs don't conflict with current prescriptions or aggravate underlying medical conditions. Medical experts can provide advice on the right dosage and duration, adjusting the herbal remedy to meet individual requirements.

Dosage Recommendations And Possible Adverse Effects

When using herbal medicines for liver and blood cleansing, dosage recommendations should be carefully considered. Although burdock root, dandelion, and milk thistle are popular herbs for liver support, taking too much of them might have negative effects.

It's critical to understand dosage to optimize benefits and reduce adverse effect risks. The necessity of moderation is highlighted by the possibility of adverse consequences such as allergic responses, gastrointestinal problems, or drug interactions.

Drug Interactions

Herbs and pharmaceuticals can interact, reducing the effectiveness of the former or producing unfavorable side effects of the latter.

People using prescription medications, particularly those for disorders of the liver or blood, should let their doctors know if they plan to use herbal medicines. This makes it possible to thoroughly evaluate any possible interactions, guaranteeing the safe and efficient incorporation of herbal remedies into the entire healthcare strategy.

CHAPTER EIGHT

HERBAL MEDICATIONS AND AMOUNTS

This guide's examination of several herbal supplements that are well-known for helping to maintain blood and liver health is one of its main features. We explore the wide variety of herbs that are well-known for having purifying qualities, offering insights into how various herbal medicines might enhance general health. We talk about the science underlying each herb and its possible advantages, from dandelion root to milk thistle.

Selecting High-Quality Supplements

Knowing how to select the best-quality goods is essential for navigating the world of herbal supplements. This section examines important variables to take into account while choosing herbal supplements, with a focus on certifications, sourcing, and purity. You can maximize the benefits of herbal medicines for blood and liver cleansing by making well-informed decisions.

Suggested Rationales

Achieving the intended health outcomes requires determining the proper dosage of herbal supplements. Here we provide advice on appropriate dosages for different herbs that are used in blood and liver cleansing. By knowing the ideal dosages, you can maximize the positive effects of these herbs while lowering the possibility of negative side effects.

Possible Relationships

It's important to be aware of any possible interactions with medications or other herbs when using supplements, just like you would with any other type. In this section, we highlight common interactions that may develop when utilizing herbal therapies for liver and blood cleansing. Being informed about potential conflicts ensures that you can integrate these natural solutions safely into your overall health regimen.

Embark on this insightful journey into the realm of herbal solutions for liver and blood cleansing, and empower yourself with the knowledge that can positively impact your well-being.

CONCLUSION

Embarking on an herbal journey for liver and blood cleansing can be a transformative step towards enhanced well-being. The incorporation of dandelion root, milk thistle, turmeric, and burdock root into one's wellness routine offers a holistic approach to supporting these vital bodily functions. As with any health regimen, it is advisable to consult with a healthcare professional before introducing new herbs, especially if there are existing health concerns or medications in play.

In summary, dandelion root acts as a liver tonic, promoting detoxification and supporting kidney function. Milk thistle, rich in silymarin, serves as a guardian of the liver, shielding it from toxins and promoting cell regeneration. Turmeric, with its golden compound curcumin, aids in liver detoxification and provides anti-inflammatory benefits. Burdock root, a blood purifier, contributes to the elimination of impurities from the bloodstream. These herbs, when incorporated thoughtfully, can play a pivotal role in maintaining optimal liver and blood health.

Encouragement For The Herbal Journey Ahead

Embarking on an herbal journey for liver and blood cleansing is a commitment to nurturing your body naturally. As you explore the benefits of dandelion root, milk thistle, turmeric, and burdock root, remember that consistency is key. Listen to your body's responses, stay informed, and consider consulting with a knowledgeable healthcare professional to tailor your herbal regimen to your individual needs. May your herbal journey be a source of vitality and well-being for years to come.

www.ingramcontent.com/pod-product-compliance
Lightning Source LLC
Chambersburg PA
CBHW060848260726
48661CB00002B/681